FAIRVIEW TRAINING
FIRST FOR TRAINING

EDUCATION AND TRAINING

DELEGATE INFORMATION PACK
(Handouts and Activities)

BLESSING ISAACKSON

FAIRVIEW TRAINING
10 Courtenay Road Wembley Middlesex HA9 7ND

Copyright © 2024 by Blessing Isaackson

All rights reserved. No part of this publication may be reproduced, distributed, or transmitted in any form or by any means, including photocopying, recording, or other electronic or mechanical methods, without the prior written permission of the publisher, except in the case of brief quotations embodied in critical reviews and certain other noncommercial uses permitted by copyright law.

For permissions requests, please contact the author.

Paperback ISBN : 978-1-7385781-0-8

Level 3 Education and Training

What are your teaching Roles?

Task 1

With regards to teaching, what are you responsible for?

INITIAL ASSESSMENT FORM   Key Task 2

| Title | |

| Name | |

| Date of Birth | |

| Address (with Post Code) | |

| Course Title | |

| Telephone number | | Mobile Phone | |

Delivery Method Required, Please Tick the box.

Blended learning ⬭   Classroom ⬭

Course Start date:

Course end Date:

Level 3 Education and Training

©Fairview Training Ltd
0208 2127315
www.fairviewtraining.com

Individual Declaration:

I confirm the accuracy of the information provided in this application form and wish to apply for the above-mentioned course in my name.

Signed

Academic Qualifications

Name of College /School	Date left	Subject studied	Grade

Vocational Qualifications

Name of college /work /establishment	Vocational Subject	Grade Gained and Year

Section 1: Background Knowledge

This section is about your roles, responsibilities, learning styles, the teaching cycle, section plan, and selecting Resources.

Have you any previous experience with regard to the contents of this section?

Yes ☐   No ☐   Little Knowledge ☐

Level 3 Education and Training — Key Task 2

Section 2: Planning and Preparation Techniques

This section is about demonstrating planning and preparation and developing and adapting a session plan to meet the learner's needs.

Have you had any experience with regard to the content of this section?

Yes ☐   No ☐   A little ☐

Section 3: Microteaching Session

The section is about teaching an inclusive microteaching section.

Have you had any experience with regard to the contents of the session?

Yes ☐   No ☐   A little ☐

Section 4: Reflective Practice

This section is about providing motivational feedback and reflecting on delivery.

Have you any previous experience with regard to the content of this section?

Yes ☐   No ☐   A little. ☐

If you have answered 'yes' or a little with regards to any of the above, could you please describe in the space provided below your experience with regard to the relevant section?

Describe your experiences concerning the sections provided above

Level 3 Education and Training — Key Task 2

> **Write what you think a prospective training provider or educational institution would not learn about the individual from this application form.**

Level 3 Education and Training — Key Task 2

Write what you think a prospective training provider or educational institution would not learn about the individual from this application form

Level 3 Education and Training — Key Task 3

> **Summarise in your own words the key aspects of legislation, the regulatory requirements, and the codes of practice relating to your own role and responsibilities.**

Level 3 Education and Training

Key Task 4

How would you promote equality and diversity within your current or (future) Teaching role?

1.

2.

3.

4.

5.

6.

7.

Level 3 Education and Training — Key Task 5

With reference to your teaching roles, list the points of referral that are available, and underneath each one describes, how they meet the needs of your learners.

1	
2	
3	
4	
5	
6	
7	

Level 3 Education and Training Key Task 6

Please circle the one response from each question that best describes your most likely action.

1. If buying a present for yourself, what will you choose?
   a. A book
   b. A CD
   c. Tools or Gadgets

2. If given a piece of equipment to operate, what would you do?
   a. Read the instructions fully first.
   b. Listen to an experienced operator give an explanation.
   c. Have a go and learn through trial and error.

3. Which of the following would you most likely say in a conversation?
   a. I see what you mean.
   b. I hear what you are saying.
   c. I know how you feel.

4. If teaching a person to do a practical task how would you prefer to do it?
   a. Give them written instructions.
   b. Show them how to do it.
   c. Tell me how to do it.

5. How would you drive a new car?
   a. Read the instructions fully first.
   b. Listen to an experienced operator give an explanation.
   c. Have a go and learn through trial and error.

6. If your friend showed you their latest electronic device, which of the following would most likely say?
   a. Show me how it works.
   b. Tell me how it works.
   C. Let me have a go with it.

7. You have taken a wrong turn and got lost. What would you do?
   a. Look at a map.
   b. Ask for directions.
   c. Try to find the route yourself.

8. You decide to cook something different and new. How do you do it?
   a. Follow a recipe.
   b. Call a friend for an explanation.
   c. Follow your instincts and taste as you cook.

9. You arrive home and find a purchase faulty. What would you do?
   a. Email the store to complain.
   b. Telephone the store to complain.
   c. Return the item immediately to the store.

10. How do you choose a holiday?
    a. Read the brochures.
    b. Listen to the recommendations.
    c. Imagine the experience

11. How do you prefer to spend any spare time you have?
    a. Visiting museums and galleries
    b. Enjoy music and conversation.
    c. Playing sports and carrying DIY.

12. You are buying a new piece of clothing for yourself. Do you?

Level 3 Education and Training

a. Look at it and imagine what it would be like.

   b. Discuss the garment with the staff.

   c. Try it on and test how it fits.

13. Mostly A's you have a visual preference   Mostly B's you have an auditory preference.   Mostly C's you have a kinaesthetic preference.

Level 3 Education and Training — Key Task 6

My own learning styles?

How does this relate to how you have enjoyed or not enjoyed learning in the past?

Level 3 Education and Training

Key Task 7

State the teaching and learning approach that you would use and then compare their strengths and limitations

Teaching and Learning approach	Strength	Limitation

Level 3 Education and Training — Key Task 8

> **Which of the following learning outcomes are SMART? Suggest alternatives if necessary**

During the session, the teacher will cover the main factors affecting the reasons for the increase in food poisoning incidents.
At the end of the session, you will be able to appreciate the importance of fire prevention.
At the end of the session, you will be able to explain the requirements for bacterial growth.
At the end of the session, you will have been given a thorough explanation of the requirements of first-aid boxes
At the end of the session, you will be able to list the factors to take into consideration when designing kitchen premises.
At the end of the session, you will be able to complete a checklist for a daily cleaning schedule.

Level 3 Education and Training — Key Task 9

Learners are required, as part of their job role, to write and send personal and business letters. Write the aims and learning outcomes of the session to teach learners how to do this

Level 3 Education and Training

Swain Analysis Form	
Name:	
Strengths	Weaknesses (1)
Aspirations (1)	Interests
Needs	
Date Produced	Target dates for attaining projects (1)

www.ingramcontent.com/pod-product-compliance
Lightning Source LLC
Chambersburg PA
CBHW042356070526
44585CB00028B/2956